The Essential Handbook On Bodyweight And Isometric Exercises For Seniors

A Comprehensive Guide To Easy, Effective Workouts For Building Strength, Improving Balance, And Enhancing Flexibility

Rose Heaney

Table of Contents

CHAPETR ONE 4
- Introduction 4
- What Are Isometric Exercises? 4
- Benefits and Advantages 5
- Safety Precautions 7
- Foundational Isometric Exercises 11

CHAPETR TWO 15
- Intermediate Isometric Exercises 15
- Advanced Isometric Exercises 19
- Isometric Exercises for Specific Muscle Groups (Upper Body Isometrics) 23

CHAPETR THREE 27
- Isometric Exercises for Functional Strength 27
- Isometric Exercises for Sports Performance Enhancement ... 30
- Resistance Band Isometrics 32
- Isometric Exercises with Gymnastic Rings 33
- Stability Ball Isometric Holds 33
- Isometric Circuit Workouts (Full Body Isometric Circuit) 35
- Targeted Muscle Group Circuits (Upper Body Focus) 36
- Lower Body Focus 36
- Core Focus 37

CHAPETR FOUR 39
- Isometric Training Programs: 4-Week Isometric Training Plan ... 39
- Advanced Isometric Workout Schedule 42

Isometric Exercises in Rehabilitation Programs 45
Injury Prevention with Isometric Training 47
Conclusion 49
THE END 52

CHAPETR ONE
Introduction

Isometric exercises are a form of strength training where the muscles contract without any visible movement in the angle of the joint. Instead of the typical repetitions and movements seen in other exercises, isometric exercises involve holding a position for a set amount of time, exerting tension against a static resistance.

What Are Isometric Exercises?

Isometric exercises target specific muscle groups and involve static contraction. Rather than moving through a range of motion, these exercises involve holding a position against resistance. For example:

- Planks: Holding a push-up position without moving the arms or legs.
- Wall Sits: Sitting against a wall with knees at a 90-degree angle.
- Static Leg Raises: Lifting and holding legs at a certain angle without movement.

Benefits and Advantages

Strength Building: Isometric exercises help build strength by engaging muscles without joint movement.

Joint Stability: They can enhance joint stability by strengthening the surrounding muscles.

Time Efficiency: Isometric exercises can be quick and effective since they engage muscles intensely without requiring a lot of time.

Safety: They are relatively low-impact and can be safer for individuals with joint issues compared to dynamic exercises.

Isometric exercises can be incorporated into a broader workout routine or used independently. They're versatile and adaptable, making them suitable for various fitness levels and goals. Additionally, they require minimal to no equipment, allowing for easy integration into daily routines.

Safety Precautions

Safety precautions are essential when performing any form of exercise, including isometric exercises. Some precautions to consider are:

Warm-Up:

- Always warm up before starting isometric exercises. Warming up helps prepare your muscles and reduces the risk of injury. Engage in light cardio or dynamic stretching to increase blood flow to the muscles.

Proper Form:

- Focus on maintaining proper form throughout the exercise. Incorrect form can increase the risk of injury and reduce the effectiveness of the exercise.

- Seek guidance from a fitness professional or use instructional videos to learn the correct technique.

Gradual Progression:

- Start with easier variations or shorter holds and gradually progress to more challenging positions or longer holds. Overexertion or pushing too hard too quickly can lead to strain or injury.

Breathing Technique:

- Maintain controlled breathing during isometric exercises. Avoid holding your breath, as this can increase blood pressure and lead to dizziness or fainting.

Listen to Your Body:

- Pay attention to your body's signals. If you feel pain, discomfort, or unusual strain during an exercise, stop immediately.

- Rest between sets or exercises to allow your muscles to recover.

Hydration and Nutrition:

- Stay hydrated before, during, and after exercising. Proper nutrition and hydration are crucial for muscle function and recovery.

Surface and Environment:

- Ensure you have a stable and safe surface to perform your exercises. Avoid slippery or unstable surfaces that could lead to slips or falls.

By following these safety precautions, you can reduce the risk of injury and maximize the benefits of your isometric exercise routine. Always prioritize safety and listen to your body's signals while exercising.

Foundational Isometric Exercises

These foundational isometric exercises are excellent for targeting various muscle groups and building overall strength. A breakdown of each exercise:

Wall Push (Isometric Push-Up)

Muscles Targeted: Chest, shoulders, triceps.

Execution: Stand facing a wall, slightly farther than arm's length away. Place your hands flat against the wall at shoulder height. Lean forward, bending your elbows to bring your chest towards the wall without actually touching it. Hold the position at the point of maximum contraction for a set time.

Plank Variations

Muscles Targeted: Core, shoulders, back.

Standard Plank: Begin in a push-up position, but with your elbows on the ground. Keep your body in a straight line from head to heels, engaging your core muscles. Hold this position.

Side Plank: Lie on your side, prop yourself up on one elbow, and lift your hips off the ground, creating a straight line from head to feet.

Reverse Plank: Sit on the ground with legs extended, hands behind you, and lift your hips off the ground, creating a straight line from head to heels.

Wall Sit

Muscles Targeted: Quadriceps, hamstrings, glutes.

Execution: Stand with your back against a wall and slide down until your knees are bent at a 90-degree angle, as if you were sitting in an imaginary chair. Hold this position for the desired duration.

Static Squat

Muscles Targeted: Quadriceps, hamstrings, glutes.

Execution: Stand with your feet shoulder-width apart. Lower your body into a squat position, keeping your back straight and knees aligned with your toes. Hold the squat position without moving for the designated time.

CHAPETR TWO
Intermediate Isometric Exercises

These intermediate-level isometric exercises offer a progression in intensity and target different muscle groups.

Push-Up Holds

Muscles Targeted: Chest, shoulders, triceps, core.

Execution: Start in a high plank position. Lower your body halfway down, keeping your elbows at a 90-degree angle, and hold this position (commonly referred to as the bottom of a push-up) without touching the ground. Ensure your body remains in a straight line from head to heels.

Isometric Lunges

Muscles Targeted: Quadriceps, hamstrings, glutes.

Execution: Step forward into a lunge position, lowering your back knee toward the ground until both knees are at about 90-degree angles. Hold this position without moving up or down, ensuring your front knee is aligned with your ankle.

Bridge Pose

Muscles Targeted: Glutes, lower back, hamstrings.

Execution: Lie on your back with knees bent and feet flat on the ground, hip-width apart. Lift your hips off the ground until your body forms a straight line from shoulders to knees. Hold this position, engaging your glutes and core muscles.

Side Plank

Muscles Targeted: Core, obliques, shoulders.

Execution: Lie on your side, prop yourself up on one elbow, and lift your hips off the ground, creating a straight line from head to feet. Hold this position, keeping your core engaged and your body in a straight line.

These exercises add complexity and challenge by requiring increased strength and stability to maintain the isometric hold. Focus on proper form and gradually increase the duration of each hold as your strength improves. Incorporating these intermediate isometric exercises into your routine can further enhance overall strength and muscle engagement.

Advanced Isometric Exercises

These advanced isometric exercises demand significant strength, stability, and control.

Planche Progression

Muscles Targeted: Shoulders, chest, core, triceps.

Execution: The planche involves holding your body parallel to the ground, supported only by your hands. There are various progressions to work towards a full planche, starting with tuck planches and advancing to straddle and full planche positions. It requires tremendous upper body and core strength.

Handstand Holds

Muscles Targeted: Shoulders, arms, core, upper back.

Execution: Assume a handstand position against a wall or freestanding. Hold your body upside down, balancing on your hands. Focus on maintaining a straight body line and engaging your core and shoulder muscles to stabilize yourself.

L-Sit Variations

Muscles Targeted: Core, hip flexors, triceps.

Execution: Sit on the floor or parallel bars and lift your legs in front of you, keeping them straight, forming an "L" shape with your body. Progress by attempting to hold the position with your hands placed beside your hips or on parallel bars.

Dragon Flag

Muscles Targeted: Core, lower back, hip flexors.

Execution: Lie on a bench or a sturdy, elevated surface, holding onto the edge for support. Lift your body off the bench, keeping it straight and rigid from head to toes, and lower your body slowly toward the ground. Hold this position and then return to the starting position.

Isometric Exercises for Specific Muscle Groups (Upper Body Isometrics)

Isometric exercises targeting specific muscle groups within the upper body, lower body, and core are:

Upper Body Isometrics(Chest and Triceps)

Isometric Push-Up Holds: Hold the bottom position of a push-up, keeping your chest and triceps engaged.

Wall Push (Isometric Push): Standing facing a wall, lean forward and hold the position with your arms at shoulder height, engaging your chest and triceps.

Shoulders and Upper Back

Isometric Shoulder Press: Push against an immovable object (like a wall) with your hands at shoulder height to engage your shoulders and upper back.

Isometric Pulling: Holding onto a sturdy bar or ledge at chest height, pull yourself towards it and maintain the position to engage the upper back muscles.

Lower Body Isometrics (Quadriceps and Hamstrings)

Static Squat: Hold a squat position at your desired depth to engage the quadriceps and hamstrings.

Isometric Lunges: Lower into a lunge position and hold it, engaging both the quadriceps and hamstrings.

Calves and Glutes

Calf Raise Hold: Rise onto the balls of your feet and hold the position at the peak of the calf raise, engaging the calves and glutes.

Bridge Pose: Lift your hips off the ground and hold, engaging the glutes and hamstrings.

Core Isometrics (Abdominals and Obliques)

Plank Variations: Standard planks, side planks, and reverse planks engage the entire core, including the abdominals and obliques.

L-Sit Variations: Lift your legs to form an "L" shape, engaging the core muscles.

Lower Back

Superman Pose: Lie face down, raise your arms and legs off the ground, and hold, engaging the lower back muscles.

Prone Bridge: Similar to the plank but resting on your forearms and toes, engaging the entire core including the lower back.

CHAPETR THREE
Isometric Exercises for Functional Strength

Isometric exercises can be tailored to enhance functional strength for everyday activities and sports performance.

Functional Isometrics for Everyday Activities

Carrying Exercise: Hold a heavy object close to your chest or at your sides for an isometric "carry" exercise, mimicking carrying groceries or a suitcase. This engages various muscle groups, including the core, arms, and shoulders.

Doorway Push/Pull: Stand in a doorway and push against the frame for isometric chest and triceps engagement. Conversely, pull against the sides of the door frame at different angles to engage the back and biceps, simulating everyday pushing and pulling movements.

Chair Squat Holds: Sit halfway down on a chair and hold the position, engaging the quadriceps and glutes, which mimics the action of sitting and standing.

Plank with Reach: While in a plank position, alternately reach one arm forward, engaging the core and stabilizing muscles, simulating the action of reaching for objects.

Isometric Exercises for Sports Performance Enhancement

Golf Swing Hold: Hold a golf club or a weighted object at the top of your backswing to engage and strengthen the specific muscles used during the swing.

Soccer Kick Hold: Hold the leg in the position just before kicking a soccer ball, engaging the hip flexors, quadriceps, and core.

Boxing Stance Isometrics: Mimic boxing stances and holds, engaging the arms, shoulders, and core muscles used during boxing movements.

Skiing/Skating Squat Holds: Hold a squat position, mimicking the body position during skiing or skating, engaging the quadriceps, glutes, and core muscles crucial for balance and stability.

These exercises help condition specific muscle groups and movement patterns relevant to various sports and everyday activities. Incorporating isometric exercises that simulate the demands of these activities can improve muscle strength, stability, and endurance, contributing to enhanced performance and reduced injury risk during these tasks.

Resistance Band Isometrics

Band Pull-Aparts: Hold a resistance band in front of you at shoulder width and pull it apart, engaging the shoulders and upper back. Hold the band at the point of maximum tension.

Band Press Holds: Secure a resistance band around a fixed object and perform a pressing motion, holding the position at the peak of the press to engage the chest and triceps.

Isometric Exercises with Gymnastic Rings

Ring Support Hold: Hold the gymnastic rings with straight arms and suspend yourself off the ground, engaging the shoulders, chest, and core to maintain stability.

Ring Row Holds: Perform a ring row and hold the top position with your chest close to the rings, engaging the upper back and arms.

Stability Ball Isometric Holds

Stability Ball Plank: Place your forearms on the stability ball and hold a plank position, engaging the core and stabilizer muscles.

Ball Squat Against Wall: Place a stability ball between your back and a wall, lower into a squat position, and hold it, engaging the lower body and core.

Using these props and tools adds instability, requiring increased muscle engagement to maintain balance and stability during the isometric holds. Remember to focus on proper form and control while using these equipment variations to maximize the effectiveness of your isometric training routine.

Isometric Circuit Workouts (Full Body Isometric Circuit)

Perform each exercise for a set duration or repetitions before moving to the next exercise. Rest for a short period between exercises if needed. Repeat the circuit for desired rounds.

Plank Hold: 30 seconds

Wall Sit: 45 seconds

Isometric Push-Up Hold: 20 seconds

Static Squat: 40 seconds

Bridge Pose: 30 seconds

Side Plank (each side): 25 seconds

Targeted Muscle Group Circuits (Upper Body Focus)

Isometric Pull-Up Hold: 20 seconds

Isometric Push-Up Hold: 20 seconds

Ring Support Hold: 30 seconds

Plank with Shoulder Taps: 40 seconds

L-Sit Hold: 20 seconds

Lower Body Focus

Wall Sit: 45 seconds

Static Lunges (each leg): 30 seconds

Calf Raise Hold: 25 seconds

Stability Ball Hamstring Curl Hold: 30 seconds

Static Squat with Resistance Band: 40 seconds

Core Focus

Plank Variations (Standard, Side, Reverse): 30 seconds each

Hollow Body Hold: 40 seconds

Russian Twists with Weight: 30 seconds

Lying Leg Raises Hold: 25 seconds

Superman Pose: 30 seconds

These circuits allow for a comprehensive workout, targeting various muscle groups in a structured and efficient manner. Adjust the durations or repetitions based on your fitness level and gradually increase the challenge as you progress. Remember to maintain proper form and engage the targeted muscles throughout each exercise in the circuit.

CHAPETR FOUR

Isometric Training Programs: 4-Week Isometric Training Plan

A breakdown of a 4-week isometric training plan and an advanced isometric workout schedule:

Week 1: Foundation Building

- **Day 1:** Full Body Isometric Circuit (Repeat 3 times)
- **Day 2:** Rest or light activity (e.g., walking, yoga)
- **Day 3:** Upper Body Isometrics (3 sets of 20-30 seconds hold per exercise)

- **Day 4:** Lower Body Isometrics (3 sets of 20-30 seconds hold per exercise)
- **Day 5:** Rest or light activity
- **Day 6:** Core Isometrics (3 sets of 20-30 seconds hold per exercise)
- **Day 7:** Rest

Week 2: Increasing Intensity

- Follow a similar structure as Week 1 but aim to increase hold times by 5-10 seconds for each exercise.
- Add a set to each muscle group or circuit routine.

Week 3: Progressive Challenge

- Incorporate variations or more challenging isometric exercises into the routines.
- Increase hold times or add a round to the circuits.
- Introduce resistance bands or stability balls for added difficulty.

Week 4: Peak Performance

- Focus on holding isometric positions with increased intensity and duration.
- Implement advanced variations of exercises to further challenge muscle endurance and strength.

- Reduce rest between sets or circuits for added intensity.

Advanced Isometric Workout Schedule

Day 1: Upper Body Emphasis

- **Planche Progression Holds:** 4 sets of 15-20 seconds
- **Isometric Pull-Up Holds:** 3 sets of 20-25 seconds
- **Ring Support Hold:** 3 sets of 30 seconds
- **Isometric Push-Up Holds:** 3 sets of 20-25 seconds

Day 2: Lower Body Emphasis

- **Wall Sit Holds:** 4 sets of 45-60 seconds
- **Single Leg Isometric Lunges:** 3 sets of 20-25 seconds per leg
- **Calf Raise Holds:** 3 sets of 30 seconds
- **Bridge Pose Variations:** 4 sets of 25-30 seconds each

Day 3: Core and Stability

- **Hollow Body Holds:** 4 sets of 30-40 seconds
- **Side Plank with Leg Lifts:** 3 sets of 20 seconds each side

- **L-Sit Variations:** 3 sets of 20-25 seconds
- **Plank with Alternating Limb Lifts:** 4 sets of 30 seconds

Day 4: Active Recovery

- Engage in light activity, stretching, or yoga to aid recovery.

Day 5-7: Repeat

- Repeat Upper, Lower, and Core Emphasis Days

Ensure to warm up before each workout and cool down/stretch after to prevent injury and aid recovery. Adjust intensity, rest, and duration based on individual fitness levels and progression. Always listen to your body and allow for adequate recovery between sessions.

Isometric Exercises in Rehabilitation Programs

Muscle Activation: Isometric exercises are often used in the early stages of rehabilitation to activate muscles without putting stress on injured joints or tissues. For example, isometric holds for the quadriceps after knee injuries.

Stability and Control: Isometric exercises help improve joint stability and control, which is crucial during the recovery phase. They can be used to target specific muscle groups around the injured area while reducing the risk of re-injury.

Gradual Progression: Isometrics allow for a controlled progression from static holds to more dynamic movements as the injury heals. For instance, transitioning from isometric leg raises to controlled leg movements after a hip injury.

Pain Management: Isometric exercises are often incorporated into rehabilitation to manage pain. They help strengthen muscles without exacerbating pain in the injured area.

Injury Prevention with Isometric Training

Strengthening Weak Areas: Isometric exercises can be used to strengthen specific muscle groups prone to injury. For instance, focusing on isometric holds for the rotator cuff muscles in the shoulders to prevent shoulder injuries in athletes.

Enhanced Joint Stability: By improving muscle strength and stability around joints, isometric training can reduce the risk of injuries related to joint instability, such as sprains or strains.

Balance and Proprioception: Isometric exercises that engage core muscles can improve balance and proprioception, reducing the risk of falls and associated injuries.

Pre-activation before Activity: Performing isometric exercises as part of warm-up routines can activate key muscles, preparing them for dynamic movements during sports or workouts, lowering the risk of acute injuries.

Conclusion

Isometric training stands as a versatile and efficient method in the realm of fitness. Its static nature allows for targeted muscle engagement without the need for elaborate equipment, making it accessible to various fitness levels and lifestyles.

By focusing on muscle contraction without joint movement, isometric exercises build strength, improve joint stability, aid in injury rehabilitation, and offer time-efficient workouts. They're adaptable, serving both as standalone routines and as complementary exercises within broader fitness regimens.

As trends evolve, isometric training continues to integrate technological advancements, offer diverse variations in equipment, and merge with other training methods, ensuring its relevance and effectiveness in the ever-evolving fitness landscape.

Whether used for rehabilitation, enhancing sports performance, preventing injuries, or simply improving overall strength, isometric exercises remain a valuable tool. As research and innovation progress, their role in promoting functional strength, convenience, and holistic fitness continues to expand, promising a future rich in versatility and effectiveness.

THE END

www.ingramcontent.com/pod-product-compliance
Lightning Source LLC
Chambersburg PA
CBHW072019230526
45479CB00008B/295